Ebook Titlᴜᴇ.

The Boiled Egg Diet: Discover How Eating Eggs Can Help Your Health And Give You The Stress-free, Fast Lane to

Weight Loss! Shed Up to 30 Pounds in 2 Weeks!

Table of Content:

Copyright Page:

only.

Introduction:

The egg diet is a low-carb diet that is associated with the Atkins diet, whose primary goal is to limit carbohydrate intake. You could have an unlimited amount of protein and fat on this diet, but your carbohydrates must be precise. Eggs are much less expensive than meat and can be used in limitless quantities while on the egg diet.

There are numerous variations of the egg diet going from just eating eggs and drinking water to using eggs as the foremost source of protein in the diet while eating other low carb foods. One prevalent variation is the egg and grapefruit diet, which, despite having no affiliation, is often referred to as the Mayo Clinic Diet.

Chapter 1

The Keto Flu:

Some folks experience flu-like symptoms when switching over to ketosis. This is called the "keto flu," and the best way to avoid this is to keep your electrolyte levels up. Drink broth or a carb-free electrolyte drink to help with the symptoms.

Know What You're Eating

Before I researched this diet, I used to try low-carb here and there. Holy craps, I now know why it never worked before; I had no clue what a net carb is! I'm pretty sure I didn't comprehend what carbohydrates were in general, but that's beside the point.

Finding your net carb is pretty simple; it's just math.

Look at the label. Take the carbohydrates (which comprises sugar), minus the fiber, and minus the sugar alcohols. It sounds complicated, but it will become second nature.

Comprehending this counting method comes in handy because foods like avocados might *seem* like they have high carbohydrates, but they also are high in fiber. So an avocado might have 13 grams of carbs,

but it has 101grams of fiber. 12-10 = 3 You can have like 10 in a day! Woohoo for guacamole! Stick with this, and you'll be in ketosis before you know it.

Sugar alcohols and fiber stop out carbs. Why? Because of science, duh. But honestly, it is because they have a negligible impact on insulin and blood sugar levels.

Some persons do have an uncanny response to sugar alcohols, so keep that in mind. Also, many nutritionists count sugar alcohols in total carbs, cutting the number in half. So if you have 7 grams of sugar alcohols, then 4 grams would count against your net carbs.

If you are feeling fine having them and don't stall your weight loss, go ahead and enjoy them! I would try to be careful when eating them though, have them at the end of your meal so you will not be tempted to overeat.

Chapter Two

How To Make Use Of Ketogenic Diet To Lose 18 Pounds Or More Instantly

You've possibly tried to lose weight several times with little to no success. Maybe you lost some weight, though it either, always came back, or your program wasn't maintainable, so you just quit.

If you're looking for a way to lose weight, especially if you need to lose 18 or more pounds, you've got to the right place.

If there's a significant thing I've discovered from my 13 years as a Holistic Nutritionist working with thousands of customers, there is A LOT of **emotional and mental pain attached to weight gain**, especially when you're weight has gotten wrong.

It might even make you angry or sad about it now, but I want to guarantee you of one thing before I get into the process:
You can either let your past pronouncements define and box you to a corner, or you could choose to move on.

Yes, your past decisions (or lack of action) have affected, maybe negatively, maybe REALLY adversely, your current situation. Moreover, your past can't be undone, BUT your past results (where you are now) CAN (where you want to be).
You can decide to move on, leave it behind you, and **start concentrating on your present!**

It's going to take time, but it's far from impossible. **I know you can do it.**
As with pretty much everything worth it, the transformation won't happen

overnight. It might take just a year or more to lose weight.

The good news? If you follow this ebook, you'll **lose weight fast**, and if you stay consistent, you'll keep losing weight, and then a year will come and go, and you would have lost a substantial amount of weight.

And **you'll keep it off!**

6 Mindset and Motivation Hacks To Help You Lose 18 Pounds or More

1.) LOSING A SUBSTANTIAL AMOUNT OF WEIGHT IS A FULL-TIME GUARANTEE

You can't be all about your weight loss goals Monday to Friday and take the weekends off. You also have to know that losing significant amounts of weight takes time and patience. Real-life is not the Biggest Loser: Healthy weight loss ranges from 0.5lbs-4lbs per week.

More than that is not sustainable and always results in relapse later on (look up the stats on how many Biggest Loser contestants gain the weight back in a year of the show!). Devotion and consistency are the names of the game!

2.) FOCUS ON PROGRESS NOT PERFECTION

As you undoubtedly know by now, significant weight loss takes time, so there will never be a chunk of time long enough where you won't have to make some hard sacrifices.

Holidays, birthdays, vacations, dinners, or nights out with friends – all of these things will come up as you are making your lifestyle changes. You will have to make sacrifices, and it will be hard. Remember your goals, communicate those goals with your friends and family. You can do it!

3.) BE OK WITH MAKING MISTAKES

I wish to remind you that "mistakes are proof you are trying." Most of the questions I receive all through the week have a common theme:
• eating something you shouldn't have
• missing workouts
• not eating enough
• eating too many "bad" carbs

Furthermore, the majority of questions or problems you have about transforming your body are about the mistakes you made. Gaffes are part of the flawed journey of weight loss, fitness, and flexible seating.

Don't dwell on your past mistakes. Don't regret your choice to skip a workout. Accept them and SELECT to make a different (better?) choice next time.

It's pretty simple when you understand YOU get to choose your action, and you get to decide how to respond to that choice/action/decision.
It's not an easy job taking charge of your mistakes, selecting to learn from them, and concentrating on how you're going to make a better choice next time. It's not easy,
BUT it's worth it, in the end.

4.) EAT RIGHT, EXERCISE, AND TRANSMUTE BECAUSE YOU LOVE YOUR BODY, NOT BECAUSE YOU HATE IT

If you are exercising and dieting since you hate your body, that's a negative place to start and will result in a negative outcome. You should be building a healthier lifestyle since you love your body and want to do what's best for it.

Be sure to set goals that aren't tied to the scale or a clothing size: Real, tangible goals like running a 6k or finally taking those dance lessons you've always wanted to care much more inspiring and fulfilling than a number on a scale or a waist circumference.

The most significant thing when trying to lose large amounts of weight is to start small and make one change at a time. Trying to make numerous changes all at once is crushing, and you will most likely fall off the bandwagon early on.
Adding a regular healthy routine every week or two that you know you will prosper at is inspiring and will make future changes more relaxed and natural.

5.) FORGET ABOUT CALORIES, POINTS, AND SCALES

You must recollect that not all calories are created equal. Five-Hundred McD's calories are not equivalent to five-hundred full food calories.

Your body NEEDS–most of your bodies are CRAVING–real food nutrients, minerals, and antioxidants.

If you don't supply your body with real food nutrients, it will keep asking for more, and hold on for (literally) dear life to whatsoever food you consume.

Do you think if you are eating 1,250 calories of crappy food, your body is going to "help" you lose weight? No way, it isn't going to happen.

The truth is you need to be eating closer to 2,050 calories of AMAZING food every day, sometimes even MORE on days that require a more metabolic function (excess stress, workout days, etc...)

More and more women are going on calorie LIMITING diets, and guess what is happening to more and more women just like YOU? You'll be GAINING more weight!

You might lose some originally, but then it comes back with a vengeance. I have the solution for you, your weight loss and food troubles, that doesn't include calorie counting, obsessing about points, or checking the scale every morning (although you'll want to because the weight will be flying off).

HERE'S HOW A KETOGENIC DIET AIDS THE WEIGHT FLY OFF (AND KEEP IT OFF)
6.) FOLLOW A RECOGNIZED HEALTH-FOCUSED SYSTEM

Alright, I must admit before I give you my formula for losing weight. I'm biased on my program because it focuses on 3 things: HEALTH, metabolism, and hormones.

If a program focuses on anything other than those 3 main things, you're doomed.

The most annoying part of working with over 10,000 individuals is that most people are trying to lose weight to get healthy when they should concentrate on getting healthy to lose weight.

That's how I'm going to assist you in beginning a ketogenic, metabolism-centered lifestyle.

Chapter 3

The 7-Step Ketogenic Plan To Lose 18 Pounds Or More.

Step 1. Skip The Exercise More Mentality

I hope I'm not starting on the wrong footing since you think I'm going to try to sell you magically "no exercise" pill.

Ultimately you'll need to start an exercise program. While it **plays a vital role in FAT LOSS, exercise plays a minor role in WEIGHT LOSS.**

If you have over 20 pounds to lose, we need to get the weight off first.

Recent research done by Current Biology took 322 adults from 6 different countries through a calorie reduction weight loss program.

They divide the groups between those that did exercise and those that did not.

Believe it or not, **adding an exercise did not play ANY chief role over calories burned or weight loss.**

And for individuals that saw alterations, they were minor at best.

When you start exercising, the first thing you'll begin doing is walking with a blend of metabolic bodyweight exercises.

Metabolic exercise makes sure you're enhancing the right fat-burning hormones and keeping your stress/fat-storing hormones low and out of the way!

Step 2. Focus On Food Quality Not Quantity

I always say, instead of suppressing your appetite, SATISFY your appetite. Too many individuals trying to lose weight are focusing on points, calories, and scale.
This isn't working, because if it were, I wouldn't have to write this eBook.

100% of the customers who desired to lose over 25 pounds and who weighed 225 pounds or more had hormonal issues that stopped them from losing weight or burning fat.

High cortisol, excess estrogen, low growth hormone, low thyroid, low testosterone, insulin resistance, and many others are likely making weight loss unbearable.
The answer?

Emphasis on NOURISHING your body with high-quality foods, macronutrients, and hormone-healing meals.

Counting calories is not only dreadful; it typically doesn't work. In addition to it, the weight continually comes back. Most of the time, even more persistent than ever before.

Step 3. Go BIG With Your Weight Loss Efforts

The bad news? Most people think it's not healthy to lose weight speedily
The truth? It's not the fact that you lose weight fast that is unhealthy, it's HOW you go about it.

The great news? **A ketogenic diet could help you lose weight quickly and in a healthy way.**

According to the newest science, militant diets win out vs. standard diets. Those who lose the most weight in the first 2-3 weeks of dieting have the most significant weight loss effects in the following year.

Thus, losing weight fast will better influence you in both the short-term and the long-term. The most operational thing you could do is truly a cold turkey method.

If you know anything about my philosophy on health and weight loss, you'll realize that I HATE short-term diets, so I say a lot about the importance of losing weight FAST.

Dropping weight fast will stimulate you to keep going. Continue making better eating choices. Keep selecting the workout over the couch.

You require a win right away if you have a lot of weight to lose, and I wish to assist you in having a FAST weight loss win.

Step 4. Balance Your Macronutrients

Now that you have decided to plan your meals (good idea!), it's about time you learn how to stabilize your meals for a fat-burning metabolism. Most folks go through specific protein and vegetables together, and that's all you require to lose weight.

While you perhaps lose weight on a protein/veggie diet, you'll end up slowing down your metabolism, AND you won't last very long eating a boring, un-enjoyable diet.

You require carbs and fat to lose fat and enhance your metabolism. The deal is in knowing which carbs and fats to incorporate in your daily eating and which ones to exclude (most of the time) from your consumption.

The most elegant approach for meal-balancing or macro-balancing that stated in this ebook starts with simplicity. Whenever you keep your meals easy, you're more likely to stick to it.

Most of the time, I propose a balanced approach to your macronutrients: carbs, proteins, and fats. Furthermore, if you're starting from scratch, I have my clients start with a Ketogenic Diet, with a focus on more fat, medium protein, and low-carb.

This form of macro-balancing steadies' insulin and leptin, the two most essential hormones for fat loss. The important thing the ketogenic diet does is changes your body from burning sugar to fat.

Step 5. Limit Your Carbs, Be Demanding With Your Protein, and Eat More Fat

You may be dealing with insulin resistance when you're overweight. I'm almost 98% sure you have insulin resistance, and I know with 100% assurance that the only way to defeat this is to do a carb-detox rather than a carb-cycle method.

Another fact with anyone overweight is they possibly aren't eating nearly enough high-quality protein. You are probably protein lacking without even knowing it.

You could even be confused as to which fats to avoid and which ones to eat. You ought to know nuts, flax oil, and olive oil are the best oils.

Furthermore, you're in for a wake-up call, because if you don't manage your carbs, increase your protein, and change your fat, weight loss will be problematic for you.

Don't worry; I'm going to make things particularly easy for you, making your weight loss seem almost effortless.
The ketosis diet includes cutting down on carbohydrates, such as rice, pasta, white bread, etc., as a low-carb diet can aid a faster weight loss process.

The ketosis diet encourages healthy fats like coconut oil, as coconut oil is rich in medium-chain triglycerides, which is enormously beneficial.

The ketosis diet also comprises protein-rich foods that can support healthy lean muscle building (metabolically active tissue), to keep you looking fit and toned.

Getting into ketosis isn't as simple as lowering your carbs and increasing fat. You need a recognized science-backed method for getting into ketosis.

Step 6. Rebuild Your Digestive System, Detox Your Liver, and Enhance Your Thyroid

Optimal digestion and incorporation of food and nutrients are vital for healthy weight loss. The hormones of the digestive tract are liable for appetite control, food digestion, nutrient absorption, and toxin removal.

Your digestive system is intensely related to your nervous system, which influences your endocrine system (hormones). If you make your stomach like a garbage dumping for low-quality foods, your hormones will repay you with weight gain.

Overconsumption of inflammatory foods can lead to a leaky gut syndrome, IBS, chronic diarrhea, ulcerative colitis, and more food intolerances. An inflamed "gut" makes it nearly incredible to have a flat stomach or engage the muscles consisting of your "core."

Optimal health and weight loss are not probable without a healthy liver. The liver is the main detoxification organ and also filters most hormones. It is responsible for 78% of T3 conversion (thyroid hormone) and offers energy in the form of glycogen. It also filters excess estrogen.

When the liver is overloaded by excess stress hormones, alcohol, processed foods, artificial sweeteners, HFCS/sugar, and an overall poor quality diet, the 2 phases of detoxification are inhibited.

The thyroid gland yields three hormones: Thyroxine (T4), Triiodothyronine (T3), and Calcitonin. T4 and T3 are what most persons think of as "thyroid hormones." These hormones play a pivotal role in your metabolism and energy control in the body.

Thyroid hormones act on nearly every sort of cell in your body to enhance cellular activity or metabolism. The breakdown of your whole body is impacted if there is a too high or too tiny thyroid hormone.

Since the thyroid hormones T3 and T4 control cellular metabolism all through the body, when there are not enough of them for any aim, this metabolic function decelerates and becomes reduced.

Since the thyroid gland regulates metabolism, there is a strong association between thyroid disease and weight. Weight gain is more severe in people with hypothyroidism due to an excess accumulation of salt and water;
weight loss is common in people with hyperthyroidism.

Step 7. Drink These 3 Drinks Every Day

Lemon Water – Drinking warm lemon water first thing in the morning is another splendid way to boost weight loss. It's also a good healthy habit to supplement your "get healthy" journey of revolution.

This drink offers **vital nutrients** for the body and is **EASY** to do. Just make sure to use a **real lemon** and not lemon juice from concentrate.
Just **squeeze 1/2 of a lemon juice inside a cup of warm water** in the morning.
Apple Cider Vinegar – Apple Cider Vinegar is one of the best liquids to heal your gut and protect your cells.

Drink this apple cider vinegar very early in the morning or request for a healthy digestive and immune system.
Ingredients:
· 9 oz. purified water
· 3 Tbsp. apple cider vinegar
· 2 tsp. raw honey (optional)
· 1/4 tsp. cinnamon (optional)
· 1/4 tsp. cayenne pepper (optional)

Metabolic Coffee/Green Tea/Yerba Mate – Coffee, green tea, and yerba mate have all been shown to be effective at motivating your metabolism and certain fat-burning hormones.

GREEN TEA INFUSION
<u>Ingredients:</u>
· Prepare a cup of green tea.
· Add 2 Tbsp. stevia or raw honey
· Add a pinch of cayenne pepper
· Add a tablespoon of ground cinnamon.

THE YERBA MATE AND HONEY ELIXIR

Yerba Mate has the "power of coffee, the health advantages of tea, and the joy of chocolate" all in one beverage. Of the seven majorly used stimulating substances in the world: coffee, tea, kola nut, and cocoa, yerba mate triumphs as the most balanced, delivering both energy and nutrition.

Ingredients:
· 2 cups yerba mate (brewed)
· 1 tsp. stevia or raw honey

THE PERFECT CUP OF COFFEE

Ingredients:
· 9 oz. of newly brewed organic coffee
· 1 Tbsp. grass-fed butter or refined coconut oil
· 1 Tbsp. MCT oil
· pinch of cinnamon

Directions:

Add all constituents to a blender and enjoy!

Step 8. Start Your Weight Loss Journey The Right Way

The 3-Week Ketogenic Diet is the best place to start your weight loss journey.
You can lose an average of 10-21 pounds in 21 days and completely love the program!
But even better than the weight loss is the feedback we get from our clients about how the program has taught them how to change their eating habits and discover a diet that works wonders for them in the long-term.

Chapter 4

How Can I Lose 18 Pounds?

The calculation for losing weight is simple: eat fewer calories than you burn. Putting this formula into practice can be perplexing, moreover. Enticements, starvation, worry, and sneaky calories disrupt your dieting efforts.

Crowded work and family timetables make fitting in exercise difficult. You are losing 18 lbs. It will take some effort and substantial lifestyle changes, but the advantages will be worth it.

Step 1

Set a genuine goal of losing just one or two pounds per week to meet your goal in nine to 18 weeks. Do not attempt crash diets or supplements that promise faster results, as these will likely fail you in the long run, warns the American Heart Association.

Step 2

Multiply your weight, in pounds, by 12 to determine the number of calories it takes to sustain your current weight, suggests Joanne Larsen, R.D. on Ask the Dietitian.

Subtract 500 to determine how many calories you need to eat daily to lose one pound per week. For instance, if you weigh 160 lbs., it takes 1,920 calories to maintain your weight or 1,420 to lose a pound per week.

Step 3

Distribute your calories over three meals and two snacks. Allocate roughly one-quarter of your daily calorie needs each to breakfast, lunch, and dinner.

Reserve the outstanding quarter for two snacks to be enjoyed during the day. For the example above, each meal would contain 360 calories and each snack about 178 calories.

Step 4

Make each meal contain a 4-oz. A portion of lean protein and a healthy carbohydrate. Pick shrimp, beans, fish, skinless poultry, extra-lean beef, tofu, or egg whites as proteins and whole-grain bread products, brown rice, sweet potatoes, quinoa, or oatmeal as healthy carbohydrates. Measure a serving as 2 cups of the grains or starchy vegetables; one slice of bread; or a serving of cereal as per the information. Eat substantial portions of watery green and orange vegetables.

Step 5

Include unsaturated fats as approximately 35 percent of your daily calories, says Larsen. Select foods such as seeds, nuts, olive oil, avocados, and salmon as your sources of fat rather than fatty meats, butter, palm oil, or fats in processed snack foods.

Step 6

Snack on fruits and low- or non-fat dairy. Choose two to three 9-oz. Servings of foods such as skim milk, cottage cheese, and plain yogurt.

Step 7

Exercise to burn off an additional 250 to 550 calories on most days to lose the 18 lbs. Faster.

Walk for an hour at a pace of 3.7 mph to burn off 279 additional calories a day, if you weigh 165 lbs, and lose another ½ pound per week. Bring your speed up to a jog of 6mph and burn 589 calories in an hour, which,

if done five times per week, can yield almost one more full pound of weight loss per week.

Follow other exercises similar to hiking, racquetball, aerobic classes, or indoor rowing and cycling to burn the same number of calories, states the expert. Write your exercise plans into your calendar and make the selection non-negotiable.

Warning:

Do not eat fewer than 1,300 calories per day as a woman or 1,600 as a man or risk nutritional deficits, irritability, and low-energy.

Consult with your doctor before starting a diet or exercise plan

Lose 37 Pound in 28 days.

Chapter 5

The Egg Diet – A Low Carbohydrate Diet:

The egg diet is a low-carb diet that is associated with the Atkins diet, whose primary goal is to limit carbohydrate intake. You could have an unlimited amount of protein and fat on this diet, but your carbohydrates must be precise.

Eggs are much less expensive than meat and can be used in limitless quantities while on the egg diet.

There are numerous variations of the egg diet going from just eating eggs and drinking water to using eggs as the foremost source of protein in the diet while eating other low carb foods.

One prevalent variation is the egg and grapefruit diet, which, despite having no affiliation, is often referred to as the Mayo Clinic Diet.

The egg diet is a low-carbohydrate, low calorie with protein-heavy food. It is intended to help in weight loss without surrendering the protein necessary to build muscles. Just as the name proposes, it underscores the egg's intake as a significant source of protein.

The egg diet is a weight loss program that requires you to eat one meal a day, and it is built around the traditional breakfast staple. It is truly a low calorie, low carbohydrate high protein plan intended to help you lose weight without losing muscle mass.

There are different forms of egg diet comprising egg only diet. In all variations of the diet plan, you would eat three meals a day with no snacks, and only water or zero-calorie beverages.

The egg diet has numerous versions, though, in each, you could only drink water or zero-calorie beverages. Food high in carbohydrates and natural sugars like most food or all bread, such as pasta and Rice, are removed from the diet, usually lasting 14 days.

You just eat breakfast, lunch, and dinner. There are no snacks, apart from water order zero-calorie drinks. Eggs are a little piece of nutrition, offering protein, Chlorine, vitamin D lutein, and many more; however, though the egg diet, on the whole, is low in carbs, which could make you hungry.

Likewise, eating the same food over and over (such as egg for breakfast) could get uninteresting for some. Which could lead to non-compliance

The egg diet has been around for quite a while. In the 1970s, the vogue newspaper circulated a famous egg and wine diet. In the internet age, it looks like the egg diet gained popularity in 2011, as the egg fest and was gotten out of the keto diet as a way to kick start delayed weight loss.

Egg diet is a nutritional livewire and provides your body with protein, fat, vitamin Phosphorus, vitamin A two B -complex vitamins that your body requires to change food into energy.

Eggs are also an exceptional source of riboflavin, selenium, and Chlorine,

There are 76 calories 5 grams of fat, 6 grams of protein, and less than 2 grams of carbohydrate in a single egg.

Chapter 6

Different Types Of Egg Diet?

There are different variations of this weight loss plan, virtually all of them.

require that you eat mainly egg-based meals, these are the most common variations

14 days' egg diet: If you pick this version of the diet program, you will eat 3 meals each day, snacks and drinks with calories are not permitted.

Each day consume one meal with eggs, though other meals can be built around different sources of lean protein like chicken or fish. To enhance the protein on your plate, you could add low carbohydrate vegetables like broccoli or spinach citrus fruits are occasionally permitted, this diet is

Sometimes known as the" boiled egg diet," and you must eat your egg hard-boiled rather than scrambled or sautéed.

Egg and grapefruit diet: This is a variation of the 14-day egg diet and continues for the same amount of time.

On this type of diet, you consume half grapefruit at each meal with your egg or lean protein; no other fruit is permitted.

Egg only diet: This type of weight loss program is mono-diet, mono diets are risky unhealthy weight loss program, where you could eat only a particular food for long periods.

Those people on these diets eat only hard boil eggs and water for 2 weeks. AS you could imagine, exercise is not suggested on this plan because of the extra fat that you are likely to witness.

Medical egg diet: This type of egg diet requires you to consume one egg and one loaf of bread three times each day, you could also eat as many fruit and vegetables as you wish.

Beverages allowed comprises water, black coffee, or other zero-calorie drink. An egg could be prepared any way you wish, as long as no calories are added.

That implies you couldn't make use of butter or oil to cook your egg. Some dieters believe that this version of the egg diet is used in medical settings to lessen a patient weight before surgery, though there is no proof to support this claim.

However, some bariatric physician put your patients on a diet before performing surgery,

it is always a liquid diet (comprising the replacement shakes), and a physician or other medical professionals monitor the program.

Keto egg diet: ketogenic diet, also known as keto diet requires that you increase your consumption of fat and put your body in the state of ketosis. This form of the egg diet suggests that you eat eggs with butter and

Cheese. To get your body to produce ketones.

The most common ratio promoted on the internet is one egg to one tablespoon of fat.

Since there is no standard egg diet, what you eat will hinge on the type you follow. In general, you could expect to eat lots of eggs, other lean protein vegetables, and some fruits.

Compliant foods:
Egg
Other lean protein like poultry and fish
Fruit like grapefruit and berries
Leafy green vegetables like spinach and Kale
Non-starchy vegetables, like broccoli mushrooms and peppers
Zero-calorie beverages like black water coffee and unsweetened tea

Non-compliant foods:

Alcohol
sugar

Refined carbohydrates such as bread and pasta
 Sweets

Milk, juice other caloric beverages

Egg diet Meal Plan:

Though there are numerous different egg diet versions, they will all work mainly the same.
You will start each day with an egg, and you will continue to eat smaller portions of lean protein all through the day.
Lean protein comprises:

 Eggs
Chicken
Turkey
Fish
 Fruits and vegetables you could eat consist of:

Grapefruit
Spinach
Broccoli
Mushrooms
Zucchini
Asparagus

In the traditional form of the egg diet, you would eat an egg or another source of lean protein like chicken or a fish at every single meal. Low- carb

Veggies or grapefruit are incorporated in breakfast and dinner. A sample meal plan would comprise of:

- Breakfast: 2 cooked eggs with one grapefruit or with 2- egg omelet with spinach and mushroom
- Lunch: 1/2 roast chicken breast and broccoli

- Dinner: 1 serving of fish and a green salad

Another form of the egg diet is the egg and grapefruit diet, in which you will consume 1 and half of a grapefruit with each meal (In place of it being optional two times a day). A new meal plan from this version of the diet would comprise:

Breakfast: 2 cooked eggs and 1/2 grapefruit
Lunch: ½ roast chicken breasts, broccoli, ½ grapefruit
Dinner: 1 serving fish and ½ grapefruit
The final type of the egg diet, which is less common is the extreme diet egg diet, in this form of the egg diet, folks only consume hard-boiled eggs and drink water for 14 days.

This diet isn't suggested as it is imbalanced and could cause starvation.

Side Effect of the egg diet:

The most notable unwanted side effects of this diet are the lack of energy several persons will feel from the depletion of the carbs; this makes it hard to exercise,
 swiftly moving to a high protein low-carb diet could also be problematic for the digestive system to adjust if you might experience things like nausea, constipation, flatulence, and bad breath.

Eggs are also very high cholesterol with 187 grams or 64% of the daily recommended value. Moreover, research has shown that it is not the cholesterol in food that we should worry about for heart health. However, there are saturated and trans fats.

A 2018 study reported that men who eat or ingest more than 7 eggs per week had a 31% higher risk of heart failure.

They also add a higher risk of ischemic stroke, ingesting 6 eggs or less per week in either men or women did not affect hemorrhagic stroke myocardial infarction or heart failures.

Since egg has no fiber, you will need to be cautious to incorporate other that do have ample amount.

This way, you won't momentarily impair bowel function or starve your healthy gut bacteria. Since this diet isn't viable, many folks return to old eating habits as soon as it is over. They would undoubtedly gain the weight back, if not even more. This could lead to yo-yo dieting, which is not very healthy for the body.

Is this diet safe:

The general agreement in the medical communities is that the egg diet isn't the safest method to lose weight.

If you are following any type of the egg diet, your calories will come in at under 1250 calories a day. According to research from Harvard medical school, it is very hazardous for women to ingest less than 1100 healthily.

calorie a day and consuming less than 1600 men unless guided by a medical professional,
Consuming up to seven eggs a week, or more in some studies appears innocuous for the general populace

With no underline side effect on cardiovascular risk. Doing so might lessen stroke risk.

A 2019 study found that even some individuals with diabetes could eat eggs more liberally than previously held about 13 per week short of worsening cholesterol level or blood sugar control.

According to one study, a high protein, low carb carbohydrate might be connected with a higher risk of cardiovascular disease.

The major disadvantage of this specific study is that it didn't control or underscore a type of carbohydrate or protein source, which could considerably impact the study outcome.

Consuming sufficient fiber everyday day is essential to nourishing gut bacteria. Americans already get far below the day-to-day suggested fiber consumption.

Since fiber is majorly found in legumes, fruit, vegetables, nuts, seeds, and whole grain, the egg diet could be worsening an already low fiber consumption.

Eggs are very convenient and resourceful; they are also very inexpensive as likened to many other protein sources and stress-free to find in any market or store.

Embrace flexibility on the egg diet: by preparing eggs in various ways with even vegetables or condiments to keep it very fascinating, there are numerous methods to prepare eggs comprising scrambled poached, hard-boiled, or fried. Omelet made with a blend of vegetables and spices will keep you from getting jaded.

Keep hard boil egg in the freezer or refrigerator: to get it on the goal.

You could also cut the egg, add them to your salad at lunchtime or make an egg salad for dinner.

Blend whole egg with egg whites: to cut calories and the saturated fat majority of the fat in the boiled egg is in the yolk, which offers about 56 calories of fat, and white protein eggs are jam-packed with -free nutrition. You would eat 4 to 6 grams of protein, 18 calories, and nearly not fat in a single egg white. Egg whites are a good source of leucine, an amino acid that could assist in losing weight.
Pros and cons
For most fad weightloss, weightloss schedule, the egg diet has significant benefits and side effects

Pros

Quick weight loss
Eggs are a nutrient-dense food

Eggs provide a good deal of protein, vitamins, fats, and minerals for about 75 calories per egg.

Cons

Deficiency of energy
Digestive issues
Might raise the cholesterol level
Crash diet leads to rebound weight gain
Some websites and videos state that you could lose 22 to 26 pounds on the 14 –day egg diet.

Moreover, these claims aren't back by any scientific study or evidence. Whereas the egg diet might promote rapid weight loss for some individuals, it is not a healthy, long-term eating plan.

Despite the promise of a rapid weight loss, the egg diet also has several drawbacks.

Lack of carbs equates to lack of energy: Since the diet is a high protein and low carbohydrate, several folks experience fatigue and lack of energy comparable to other low-carb plans.

Eggs could make you gassy: Several individuals on the egg diet experience gas, constipation, nausea, and bad breath, which are all known side effects of a high protein diet. You could battle digestive problems by getting more fiber from vegetables in your diet and drinking more water.

High cholesterol food can lead to heart disease:
Eggs are high cholesterol food, which has been associated with increased

blood cholesterol levels and heart disease. Furthermore, the novel research called this into question. According to a research 2019 review article distributed in the journal nutrition,

the connection between egg and heart disease is unsubstantiated. Another 2019 review in the Canada journal of diabetes states that consumption of 7-13 eggs per week doesn't affect total cholesterol LDL cholesterol cluster lights fasting.

Glucose, insulin, triglycerides, or c-reactive protein level all indicators of a heart, if you are at risk of heart disease talk to your physician before starting the egg diet.

Short term weight loss is difficult to endure:
like the most diet that promises swift weight loss over a short time, the egg

diet isn't viable, and pounds lost are expected to be recouped. ever since you don't

Learn any healthy eating habits on this program, such as portion control, balanced meal planning, or mindful eating. It is probable to return to the food habits that triggered the weight gain in the first instance.

The egg diet is too restrictive: Though you might be able to wriggle through two weeks of just eating one food(only a small number of food), the hunger and uneasiness you are most likely to encounter will be overwhelming. Several dieters are bingeing on junk food or just leaving the diet completely.

Chapter 7

How it compares:

Although egg is jam-packed with healthy nutrients, your body requires more than the nutrients in the egg to function efficiently; for instance, fiber enhances healthy digestion, and you are not likely to get the fiber you require when you are on this diet.

Whenever we consume a wide range of nutritious food, it helps us sustain good health and the right weight.

Most kinds of egg diets are not well rounded enough to provide your body with the energy it needs to function correctly. if you are to follow the egg diet correctly,

You would likely lose a few pounds possibly up to 6 pounds in a week and a few more the subsequent week. However, the weight you will lose would mostly be water weight, not fat, and that is an essential drawback to keep in mind.

Although the egg diet may offer quick weight loss to assist you in reaching a short-term goal, it is not very healthy or sustainable in the long run?

USDA recommendation:

The U.S. Department of Agriculture USDA directory guidelines compose of suggestions and tips for a healthy balanced diet; the following nutrient-dense food is suggested as part of a healthy diet.

Vegetable and dark leafy greens (kale spinach, broccoli to swiss chard and green beans
Fruits (apple melon berries)
Grains (brown rice oats quinoa)
Lean meat (chicken breast, fish and turkey breast)
Beans and legumes (all beans lentils and peas)
Nuts and seeds (almond, walnuts sunflower seeds)
Dairy (reduced fats milk, cheese, yogurt)
Oils (olive oil, avocado oil)
The egg diet does not offer to encompass nutrition and doesn't meet up the USDA guidelines it is not well known as a very healthy long-term diet

Similar diet

Much like the egg diet, these other vogue diets restrict the menu to a particular food. Whereas each plan promise you will drop pounds instantly, they are unlikely to offer long-term viable weight loss.

Cabbage soup diet: The primary focus of the diet is a home-based soup eating many times a day. The diet also composed of other foods that could be eaten on particular days.

Juice Cleanse: A 3 day- fast, the juice cleanse proposes drinking raw, an organic liquid made from fruits and vegetables numerous times a day. Food, other than that which is juice, is not permitted.

Grapefruit diet: A new diet with a potential of rapid weight loss, the grapefruit diet is a 10-day plan that that permits eating grapefruit or sipping grapefruit juice with every other meal.

The three-day military diet: This plan offers a particular list of food to eat on special days comprising things like two hotdogs without buns, 6 saltine crackers, and a cup of vanilla ice cream.

Despite the name, the diet is not restricted to 3 days or a link to the military; you could eat specific foods for 3 days with calories limited 1600 a day on the 4 off days.

M- plan: On this diet, the M represents mushroom, and you could swap one meal a day for 2 weeks with a low-fat or fat-free mushroom made dish. it doesn't otherwise check calorie or other food groups, however, swapping out meat for mushroom

.

The truth is that this diet will not lead to long-term changes that enhance your health.

Of lessen daily calorie consumption to assist you to lose weight.

The boiled egg diet demand that you eat two or three eggs per day at least Do you like eggs

Do you love eggs? Thus, the boiled egg diet might be for you, particularly if you wish to lose weight.

Chapter 8

What is a Boiled egg diet?

A boil egg diet is a form of Diet that Focuses on egg precisely on hard- boil an egg, you consume a minimum of two to three eggs each day, and you don't even have to infuse them into every meal, why would somebody want to consume this way?

It has a bit of celebrity support Nicole Kidman supposedly ate only hard-boiled egg before staring in cold mountain according to vogue newspaper,
yes, was the nice husband of Charley Saatchi-, the ex-husband of Nigella Lawson, the creator of the ad agencies Saatchi& Saatchi has also done the boiled- egg diet on boiler guys

according to some publication like Daily independent.

How does boiled egg diet work?

According to the expert boiled egg diet, there are numerous versions of the boil- egg diet that is the fastest and easiest way to lose weight. We will jump into different options

Breakfast: at least three eggs and one piece of fruit or low-carb vegetable
Lunch: Egg or lean protein and with low carb vegetable
Dinner: Egg or lean protein and low carb vegetable

Is the boiled egg diet right for you?

Generally, this diet comprises healthy food though it is not a balanced diet, the boiled egg diet is very restrictive, extremely low calorie and faddish, I don't feel you should be on a diet that requires an obsession with one food says an expert.

The root of the diet- the egg is a food that is healthy for you merely not as your only or significant food.

The American Health Association states that one egg or two egg whites a day could be a portion of a healthy diet. The egg makes a splendid breakfast. A hard-boiled is a nutritional snack though I think that eating a range of food is more robust means to eat, says the expert.

The unique thing about the egg is that they are high in protein. one great boiled egg gives 72 calorie system of protein 7 gram of fat 0.4 for gram of carbohydrates 0 g fiber

Egg a complete protein and comprise nutrients such as vitamin C and Chlorine Amy Shapiro, the founder, and director of Essential nutrition in New York City,

(A whole protein is one that has all the essential amino acids according to the U.S. Food and Drug Administration.

Chlorine is a nutrient that helped produce neurotransmitters that control memory and moods amid other functions, according to data from National Institute of health.

Though some past studies have associated breakfasts high in protein that comprises egg with assisting dieters of losing some pounds as associated, there is nothing enchanted about egg for weight loss says, Shapiro.

Side effects of eating mostly boiled egg:

This diet is low calories and controls many high-fiber foods such as whole grains and beans; because of that, you could miss the spot on fiber if you aren't very careful.

It is suggested that men age 50 and younger get at least 40 grams of fiber, and women get at least 27 g fiber. Go too low, and you might be at risk of constipation mainly if you consume only eggs, As egg has zero grams of fiber.

Is It Safe To Follow The Boiled Egg Diet:

if you are on a boil egg diet for a short period, you are mostly healthy; it is not likely to cause any problems. I see it as a special diet. It is merely something to attempt when you wish to see speedy results,

and you are ok with Feeling limited for a short period, said Shapiro, the nutritionist.

She opines that this diet takes its hints from the 1960s, which is considered ladylike and modest to limit yourself, she stated. Hence, this is not a healthy headspace to be in.

There is unending confusion about whether an egg is suitable for you as it has dietary cholesterol. Each egg has 185 mg of cholesterol, according to the USDA. research widely distributed in June 2019 in the journal of America Medical Association stated that each additional

320 g of dietary cholesterol eating per day was connected with 18 to 19 percent increase risk correspondingly of cardiovascular disease and death from any source. Furthermore, another research was distributed in July

2019 in the American Journal of Nutrition, stated that cholesterol is less dangerous in adults with prediabetes, type2diabetes. The authors said that partakers.

Who consumed a high egg diet for 4 months didn't witness changes in blood lipid levels or indicators of inflammation (which would point to a change in cardiovascular health. As compared to those on the low- egg diet.

Scientists have defined a high –egg diet as eating 13 or more eggs per week, though they said dieting a low-egg diet involves eating fewer than three eggs per week.

Though many people are worried over dietary cholesterol, the limit was eliminated from the 2017 to 2021 nutritional plans,

Moreover, the guideline state that this change does not suggest that does not state that dietary cholesterol is no longer essential as a condition when building healthy eating pattern going on to advise individual to ingest as little dietary cholesterol as probable.

Eggs are also marked for their saturated fat content. Each large egg has 1.7 g of saturated fats; the guide suggests capping daily ingestion saturated fat at less than 11% of a calorie per day for ideal heart health.

Are egg safe for people with diabetes to eat

Thus, are eggs good or bad for you? Taking into cognizance of the study as a whole, Shapiro stated that it is saturated fat in food that increases cholesterol, not primarily dietary cholesterol.

One more time, it is simple carbohydrates and sugar in food that raise cholesterol and triglycerides. I wouldn't bother about eating hard-boiled eggs every day she opines. However, if that is the bulk of what you are taking that saturated fat could pile up.

Shapiro gives her customer the go-ahead to eat 3 eggs per day; however, this health advice look differs yearly according to other health organizations, To be on the safer side, if you have diabetes or any risk factors for heart disease, consult your healthcare team, how many eggs are right for you to eat.

What to Eat and Avoid:

According to many experts, the following food is suggested on the boiled- egg diet to avoid; the eating plan is very stringent. You are not to go off track from this list.

- Skinless Poultry

- Egg
- Fish
- Lean beef
- Beef and pork
- Low carb vegetable comprising leafy green, such as Kale, collard

green, spinach with mustard green, Zucchini, and pepper.
- Local carb fruit like tomato, oranges, lemons, limes, watermelon, strawberries cantaloupes, and peaches, and grapefruit.
- Calorie-free drink such as plain water and sparkling water
- Butter

.

Takeaway:

The egg can be a beneficial protein; however, it should not be the only food an individual eats.

The egg diet might lead to weight loss first; moreover, it is not a balance or safe weight loss or weight loss plan in the long term. As soon as a person returns to their regular eating pattern, they may regain the weight in some weeks.

Moreover, any limiting diet can restrict a person's consumption of essential nutrients.

In the long run, there are healthier ways to lose weight than the egg diet. Making viable changes, like cutting out treated food, reducing meat and dairy consumption and eating more fruits and vegetables could help a person sustain a healthy weight over time.

The long-term solution to improving health and perhaps losing weight include the Mediterranean diet and the dash diet.

Q

Will an egg raises my cholesterol level ?:

A

Research is diverse on this topic. Moreover, the present suggestions have removed the above dietary guidelines to ingest no more than 322 mg of cholesterol every day.

Scientists have stated that trans and saturated fat play a more vital role in the development of heart disease over cholesterol. Experts still advise individuals to restrict cholesterol to sustain a healthy eating pattern.

As specified before, the egg has about 76 calories and 14 different vitamins and. There is an enormous 8 grams of protein in a hard-boiled egg, and the low-calorie option is ideal for weight loss.

.

An egg has vitamin, phosphorus, vitamin B12, and essential amino acid. Egg also has about 15% of your daily riboflavin consumption; it also comprises folate, iron, vitamin B6, and zinc. of four late-comer iron former vitamin C and zinc.

Application of dietary practices for weight loss:

As stated before, you shouldn't rely majorly on any food for your nutrition. Our body needs different kinds of food to sustain optimum Wellness. The extreme form of the boiled –egg diet is limiting and only permit dieters to eat boiled egg and water. Furthermore, this is risky and unnecessary to incorporate varieties of crucial food.

Chapter 9

Egg Diet Plan: Sample meal plan for weight loss:

We take the best part of the boiled egg diet and make it better and very viable.

Diet Meal Plan:

Breakfast:3 eggs (any style)

Breakfast: 3 eggs (any smooched) + 1 piece of fresh fruit (such as apple, pear, berries) + 1 cup of whole-grain toast + 1-3 teaspoon butter + 1 glass of drinking water

Lunch: 3-5 ounces of lean protein (such as. chicken, tuna) + 1 cup of simmered vegetables + 1/2 cup brown rice + 7oz yogurt for dessert + 1 glass drinking water

Dinner: 3-5 ounces of bony protein (like 99% bony ground turkey + 1/2 cup fajita veggies + 1 whole-grain tortilla + 1 serving of fresh fruit for dessert (such as. 3/5 cup blueberries)

Snack Ideas (eat 0-2 snacks per day): 9oz low-fat or nonfat milk, 1 low-fat or nonfat string cheese, 1/5 cup nuts, 1 serving of fruit, 2 cups raw veggies with 3Tbsp of dip

Other diets for weight loss:

Use Veggies to your benefit:

With the exclusion of potato, corn, and peas, local –carb veggies like lettuce, spinach, Kale, peppers, and eggplant are a low-calorie food that could assist you to bulk your meals.
Put these veggies on your plate to make you jam-packed for minimal calories.

It is essential to drink sufficient water to boost your protein fiber intake during the boil egg diet. For those who usually don't eat fruit and vegetable, add them slowly and stay hydrated to stop constipation.

Also, if you are beginning to increase your protein consumption, hydration is vital. This is because a high level of protein could also constipate you or demanding a significant organ.

Typically, water is crucial for any weight loss plan full. Water is useful in flush out your kidney, keeps your skin and brain healthy.
Practice calorie control:

When beginning to lose weight, calorie control is essential.
Furthermore, for precise suggestions, see a certified dietician; moreover, according to Harvard medical school,

common women should not consume fewer than 1300 and men, not more than 1600 calories a day.

They are ingesting less than these thresholds could rob you of vital nutrients.

These days, there are different apps to track your calorie consumption to learn about your calorie content.

Learn about portion size:

Portion sizes of food could help you know if you are ingesting too much or too little of a particular food item. Make use of portion size to check yourself and as a way to make changes to your diet. Portion sizes are typically compared to everyday household items for easy visualization.

Know some stress-free weight loss hacks:

Who doesn't love to be told some guidelines for Success? These are some tried-and-true techniques to reduce your calorie intake.

- In place of two pieces of bread for a sandwich, use one slice of bread for an open-faced sandwich.
- Swop bread with a lettuce wrap for small tortilla
- Swop established Rice for cauliflower rice
- In place of candy or sweets, go for fresh fruits
- In place wheat pasta, go for veggies noodles or bean pasta,
- Swap soda, go for seltzer water with non-caloric flavoring

- In place of ice cream, select protein-packed Greek yogurt
- When eating oily food (like pizza) take a napkin and immerse it in grease

This modest switches could lessen the number of calories you ingest. Try to implement 2 to 3 of these hacks nowadays.

Brilliant Ways To Make Eggs (impeccable Hard-boiled eggs) :

Have you ever tried to boil an egg and get upset? Since the shells stick to the egg, you aren't alone on this. Don't waste your eggs, mainly if you have spent on the omega 3 rich egg; We have some tips on how to boil egg make them ideal for your home.

These are the ways To make perfect hard-boiled egg at home:

1Making use of safety pin, punch a hole at one end of each egg. This would assist the shell to come off later.

2 Place your egg in a pot and cover it with cold water,

3 Turn the burner on high and bring it to a boil.

4 After the water starts boiling, allow eggs to boil in water for about 12 minutes for (softer yolks, boil for less than 12 minutes, for firmer yolks, boil more than 12 minutes.

5 After this, turn off the burner and instantly drain the pot.

6 Fill the container with cold water again to cover the egg.

7 Because of the egg and pot's temperature, It's unavoidable that your egg
will become warm again. You don't want; you want cold egg in cold

water. Put some ice cube into water. Allow the eggs to sit for 15 to 33

minutes in the cold water.

Whenever you come back to peel the egg, the shell will come right off, leaving you with no wasted egg and flawlessly hard-boiled egg every time!

Change it up:

To shake things up, these are some of the things you could do with hard boil egg

Slice up and use as a salad icing
Squash up and put on toast or on a club sandwich
Chop up to use egg salad or pasta dishes

Magnificently chop and Put over fresh or boiled vegetables.

Add to Rice, quinoa, or couscous.

Can I cook the egg in another way?

Yes, you could typically cook in other ways; there are few methods you could ponder about.

Scramble egg: Add onion, garlic, fresh parsley, tomato and spinach, and many more. For reducing calories, use a cooking oil spray in place of a liquid or butter.

Fried egg: Once more, pile on the veggies make use of a cooking spray always to deep-fry

Egg salad: for a healthy switch with good fats, make egg salad with avocado in place of mayonnaise, Add in some celery and onion for flavor and fiber.

Deviled egg: in place of Mayo (and less guilt) select an avocado

Not minding how an egg is prepared, try to remember that method of cooking and added components. Will all play into the calorie count of the meal. The controlling portion will assist you in enjoying all types of eggs while trying to lose weight.

Spice up your egg:

Eating a hard-boiled egg by itself gets very old. These are some yummy proposal to spice up your egg.

- Mustard (particularly coarsely ground mustard or Dijon mustard)
- Salt and pepper
- Tamari or soy sauce
- Hummus
- Hot sauce

Although egg is excellent, that they could bring, make your diet varied and well rounded, so that you could stick to your eating plan for a long time— the button and apologies for the bottom line on the boiled egg diet.

Chapter 10

THE EGG DIET 28 DAY

If you wish to lose pounds in a hassle-free and relaxed way without sacrificing something? Then, this Egg diet 28 day is an excellent assistance for you to lose up to 37 pounds in 28 days.

Recall to: Get ready to start eating eggs (boiled). Eradicate Junk food. Lessen the amount of salt. Sugary drinks or alcohol must be shunned, mainly processed sugars.

FIRST DAY (First Week)
On Breakfast
- 1/2 Orange or Grapefruit

- 1 or 2 Boiled Eggs

2. Lunch: Try to eat as much of one fruit that you like, see fruits below.

- Orange, Strawberry, Pears, Apples, Plums, Cantaloupe, Watermelon

3. Dinner – Chopped meat only wholly fat-free, Cut or Ground

* mutton or lamb are not permitted

DAY 2

1. Breakfast

- 1/2 Orange or Grapefruit
- 1 **or** 2 Boiled Eggs

2. Lunch – Sautéed or boiled chicken only. *, remove the skin.

3. Dinner – 2 boiled eggs, green salad, One slice of toast or pita and one orange or grapefruit

Day 3

1. Breakfast

1/2 Orange or Grapefruit

1 **or** 2 Poached Eggs

2. Lunch :
– One tablespoon of fat-free cream cheese, A portion of toast with tomato.
3. Dinner :
– Topped meat (cut or ground), green salad(lettuce, tomato, green pepper, carrots, cucumber

DAY 4
1. Breakfast
½ Orange or Grapefruit -
1-2 Cooked Eggs -
2. Lunch – Get as many as one fruits that you relish, select one of the fruits below.
Orange, Strawberry, Pears, Apples, Plums, Cantaloupe, Watermelon and mango
3. Dinner – Chopped meat (cut or ground), green salad(lettuce, tomato, green pepper, carrots, cucumber)

DAY 5
1. Breakfast
½ Orange or Grapefruit -

1-2 Simmered Eggs -

2. Lunch – 2 simmered eggs, broiled vegetables(zucchini, squash, spinach, carrots, green beans, or peas)

3. Dinner – Sautéed Fish, Shrimp, or 1 can of tuna in water. (Choose 1 of the 3)

DAY 6
1. Breakfast
½ Orange or Grapefruit -
1-2 Cooked Eggs -

2. Lunch – Get as much of one fruit that you adore, select one of the fruits below.

Orange, Strawberry, Peas, Apples, cucumber, Cantaloupe, Watermelon

3. Dinner – Sliced meat (cut or ground), green salad (lettuce, tomato, green pepper, carrots, cucumber)

DAY 7
1. Breakfast
½ Orange or Grapefruit -
1-2 Cooked Eggs -

2. Lunch – Topped or roasted chicken. Seared or boiled vegetables (zucchini, squash, spinach, carrots, green beans, or peas), and one orange or grape fruit.

3. Dinner – Heated or boiled vegetables (zucchini, squash, spinach, carrots, green beans, or peas)

DAY 8 (Second week)
1. Breakfast
½ Orange or Grapefruit -
1-2 Heated Eggs -

2. Lunch – 2 heated eggs and one orange or grapefruit.

3. Dinner – 2 simmered eggs and one orange or grapefruit

DAY 9
1. Breakfast
½ Orange or Grapefruit -
1-2 sauteed Eggs -

2. Lunch – Meshed meat (cut or ground), green salad(lettuce, tomato, green pepper, carrots, cucumber).

3. Dinner – 2 heated eggs and one orange or grapefruit
enchanting

DAY 10

1. Breakfast

½ Orange or Grapefruit -

1-3 Poached Eggs -

2. Lunch – Seared meat (cut or ground) and cucumbers. (any quantity you want)

3. Dinner – 2 heated eggs and one orange or grapefruit

DAY 11

1. Breakfast

½ Orange or Grapefruit -

1-2 Simmered Eggs -

2. Lunch – 2 seared eggs, one tablespoon of fat-free cream cheese, and boiled or steamed vegetables.

3. Dinner – 2 chopped eggs and poached or cooked vegetables

DAY 12

1. Breakfast
½ Orange or Grapefruit -
1-2 cooked Eggs -
2. Lunch – Seared or fried fish or shrimp.
3. Dinner – 2 boiled eggs

DAY 13
1. Breakfast
½ Orange or Grapefruit -
1-2 Simmered Eggs -
2. Lunch – Sliced meat, tomato, one orange, or grapefruit.
3. Dinner – Blend of fresh fruit (orange, cantaloupe, plum, apples, and watermelon)

DAY 14

1. Breakfast
½ Orange or Grapefruit -
1-3 Cooked Eggs -
2. Lunch – Meshed or cooked chicken (skin detached), tomato, and one orange or grapefruit.
3. Dinner – Chopped or cooked chicken (skin detached), tomato, and one orange or grapefruit.

DAY 15 (Third Week)
1. Breakfast
½ Orange or Grapefruit -
1-2 poached Eggs -
2. Lunch – Any fruits, any quantity, and time (deprived of grapes, mango, dates, bananas, and figs).
3. Dinner – Any fruits, any quantity, and time (without grapes, mango, dates, bananas, and figs).

DAY 16
1. Breakfast

½ Orange or Grapefruit -

1-2 Boiled Eggs -

2. Lunch – Any cooked or steamed vegetables and any green salad, any quantity, and time.

3. Dinner – Any boiled or steamed vegetables and any green salad, any amount, and time.

DAY 17

1. Breakfast

½ Orange or Grapefruit -

1-3 Poached Eggs -

2. Lunch – Any form of fruit and poached or steamed vegetables with any green salad, any quantity, and time.

3. Dinner – Any fruit and cooked or steamed vegetables with any green salad, any amount, and time.

DAY 18

1. Breakfast

½ Orange or Grapefruit -

1-2 Heated Eggs -

2. Lunch – Topped or sautéed fish or shrimps any quantity, anytime with lettuce.

3. Dinner – Sliced or simmered fish or shrimps any number, anytime with lettuce

DAY 19

1. Breakfast

½ Orange or Grapefruit -

1-2 simmered Eggs -

2. Lunch – Any fruit and boiled or steamed vegetables with any form of green salad, any quantity, and time.

3. Dinner – Any fruit and boiled or steamed vegetables with any green salad, any number, and time.

DAY 20 & 21

1. Breakfast

½ Orange or Grapefruit -

1-2 poached Eggs -

2. Lunch – One kind of fruit is allowed, and you have to select one of the following (apples, pears, plums, apricots, & guava) for two successive days in any quantity and at any time.

3. Dinner – One sort of fruit is allowed, and you have to select one of the following (apples, pears, plums, apricots & guava) for two successive days in any quantity and at any time

DAY 22 (Last Week)

During this week, you can have only the stated quantities for each day, but you can eat. During this week, you can have only the amounts reported

for each day, but you can eat it in any arrangement or at any time of the day as you wish. It in any blend or at any time of the day as you love.

* 5pieces of capped meat (no fat) or 5 pieces of boiled meat or ¼ of boiled or meshed chicken (no skin).
* 4 tomatoes and 5 cucumbers
* One can of tuna in water
* two pieces of browned bread or ¼ crisped Arabic bread (pita)
* Two oranges or grapefruit

DAY 23

During this week, you can have only the stated quantities for each day, but you can eat. During this week, you can have only the specified amounts for each day,
but you can eat it in any blend or at any time of the day as you wish. It in any combination or at any time of the day as you want.

* 3 pieces of sautéed meat no more than 19 ounces or 250 grams.
* 4 tomatoes and 5 cucumbers
* One part of toast or ¼ toasted Arabic bread (pita)

* One fruit (apple, pear, guava, or two slices of cantaloupe or watermelon)
*One orange or grapefruit

DAY 24
You can have only the definite quantities for each day during this week, but you can eat. During this week, you can have only the specified amounts for each day, but you can eat it in any combination or at any time of the day as you wish. It in any mixture or at any time of the day as you want.
* Two tablespoons of fat-free cream cheese.
* Two can of tuna in water
* 3 tomatoes and 3 cucumbers
* One piece of toast or ¼ toasted Arabic bread (pita)
* One orange or grapefruit

DAY 25

This week you can have only the definite quantities for each day, but you can eat. You can only have the exact numbers for each day during this week, but you can eat it in any combination or at any time of the day as you demand.

It in any combination or at any time of the day as you desire.

* ½ cooked or grilled chicken (no skin).
 * 3 tomatoes and 4 cucumbers
 * One piece of toast or ¼ crisped Arabic bread (pita)
 * One fruit (apple, pear, guava, or one slice of cantaloupe or watermelon)
 * One orange or grapefruit

DAY 26

Throughout this week, you can have only the definite quantities for each day, but you can eat it in any combination or at any time of the day as you wish. It in any combination or at any time of the day as you want.

* 3 boiled eggs.
* One head of lettuce and 4 tomatoes
* One orange or grapefruit

DAY 27
During this week, you can have only the specified quantities for each day, but you could eat it in any combination or at any time of the day as you wish.
* 2 chicken breast (chopped or boiled – no skin)
* One teaspoon of fat-free cream cheese.
* 3 tomatoes and 23cucumbers
* One piece of toast or ¼ roasted Arabic bread (pita)
* One orange or grapefruit

DAY 28

All through this week, you can have only the specified quantities for each day, but you can eat it in any combination or at any time of the day as you wish.

It in any combination or at any time of the day as you want.
 * Two tablespoons of fat-free cream cheese.
 * two can of tuna in water
 * 2 tomatoes and 2 cucumbers
 * One piece of toast or ¼ cooked Arabic bread (pita)
 * One orange or grapefruit

If you've followed this diet precisely, I'm sure you're happy with your results. Make sure to share this with your friends and family members. This is a proven system that will work for anybody looking to lose weight in a short period.

Conclusion on the Egg diet:

As we have discussed, the boiled egg diet has become a popular weight-loss fad, with us with that is very limiting and not viable for a very long time.

Now that you know what dietician analysis of the diet, you have the tool you need to make a better, more workable weight loss plan.

While egg can be part of a healthy weight loss diet and make sure your egg diet menu is well versed.

Optimistically, the egg diet now appears a little less intricate.

It should be clear that this diet is also precious. It doesn't matter whether you

want to lose weight, enhance your metabolism, or help with diabetes.
An egg diet can be beneficial for many individuals.

It might be hard at first; if you stick with it, you'll gain the rewards in due course. And remember, this isn't some crazy theory.

There could be part of a healthy weightloss, weightloss that make sure your egg diet menu is well branded.
We gave easy guidelines, such as drinking sufficient water, selecting lean protein, quoting, and piling up the vegetable.

When it comes to long-term and viable weight loss plans, choose an eating plan that focuses on healthy foods, and control calories; honey is non-restrictive.